I0025569

# My Childhood Cut Short

*Surviving Leukemia and Finding Purpose Beyond Pain*

# My Childhood Cut Short
### Surviving Leukemia and Finding Purpose Beyond Pain

## Tony Garcia

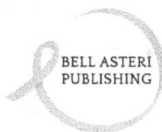
BELL ASTERI
PUBLISHING

My Childhood Cut Short
*Surviving Leukemia and Finding Purpose Beyond Pain*
Copyright ©2026 by Tony Garcia

Author: Tony Garcia
Editor: Mariah Forster Olson
Foreword by Dana-Susan Crews
Content Contributions by Bell Asteri Foundation

All rights reserved. No part of this publication may be reproduced, stored in a retrieval system, or transmitted in any form or by any means - for example, electronic, photocopy, or recording - without the prior written permission of the publisher. The only exception is a brief quotation in printed reviews.

The opinions expressed by the author are not necessarily those of Bell Asteri Publishing & Enterprises, LLC.

Published by Bell Asteri Publishing & Enterprises, LLC
209 West 2nd Street #177
Fort Worth TX 76102
www.bellasteri.com

Published in the United States of America

ISBN: 978-1-957604-84-8 (paperback)
ISBN: 978-1-957604-85-5 (hardcover)

# Contents

Tony Garcia

I dedicate this book to my parents, Sylvia Wilmot and A. Hector (Buddy) Garcia, whose courage, prayers, love, and unwavering support helped save my life. To my siblings, Rosalie Keszler, Patricia Garcia-King, and Buddy Garcia, who were forced to grow up in the whirlwind of childhood cancer, this is also for you.

And to every childhood cancer warrior fighting to survive each day, you are seen, you are brave, and you matter. Someday, we will win this war on childhood cancer.

Tony Garcia

# Foreword

by Dana-Susan Crews
Founder, the Bell Asteri Foundation

*I* will never forget the moment I met Tony Garcia. I was new in town, having just moved up to North Texas from Southeast Texas. My children were both in college, and I wanted to get involved in local charities with a mission to cure cancer. For many years, I had been deeply involved in cancer-related philanthropy, particularly with blood cancers and childhood cancers. Through MD Anderson Cancer Center and Blood Cancer United (formerly the Leukemia & Lymphoma Society), I had helped raise funds, awareness, and support for research and patients. Cancer had long been close to my heart, and I felt called to continue that work.

About a week after my move, I received a message on LinkedIn from a recruiter asking if I would be interested in a development position with the American Cancer Society. I was surprised. I had never seriously considered ACS before, largely because of a common yet incorrect assumption that they did not invest significantly in pediatric cancer research. Like many others, I believed their focus was elsewhere. What I did not yet know was just how wrong that assumption was and how profoundly that misunderstanding would soon be corrected.

I agreed to an interview at the North Texas chapter of ACS. When I walked through the doors, I was greeted warmly by Tony, who had already been working there for several years. We chatted briefly, exchanging the kind of polite conversation that leaves a smile in your heart. Tony was immediately kind, gracious, and genuine. I remember thinking, almost instantly, "This may be one of the nicest people I've ever met." There was something steady and sincere about him, a warmth that made me feel welcome without effort. At the time, I had no idea that Tony was a long-time childhood cancer survivor.

The interview process moved quickly, and I soon accepted the position. Tony and I became coworkers, and in time, friends. As I learned more about him, I was struck by something extraordinary. Tony had endured brutal leukemia treatments as a toddler and young child, treatments from an era when survival rates were painfully low. Children diagnosed in the early 1970s rarely lived to adulthood. In fact, Tony was the longest living childhood cancer patient I had ever met.

Over the following year, I learned more about the depth of his journey. About the pain, the resilience, and the quiet strength that had shaped him. I have always been fascinated by a particular truth. Some of the strongest, kindest, and most compassionate people in this world are those who have carried the greatest burdens. Tony exemplifies this in every way.

You would never know how much he had endured unless he chose to tell you. He was not someone who sought attention or sympathy. He did not wear his suffering on his sleeve. Instead, he lived a life defined by generosity, humility, and unwavering goodness. Tony focused outward, on how he could help, encourage, and uplift others. He worked tirelessly to raise awareness and funding to fight cancer, particularly for those who were still in the middle of their battle.

He did not complain when the days were long or the work was

hard. He showed up. He smiled. He encouraged those around him. He worked harder than anyone else and consistently went the extra mile, not because he had to, but because he cared deeply. His compassion was not performative. It was lived out daily through action.

My time at the American Cancer Society was not long. After some personal circumstances required my attention, I resigned my position. Not long after, Tony also resigned to pursue another opportunity. But his commitment to the cause never wavered. He continued to volunteer with organizations like Blood Cancer United, raising both awareness and funds for research and patient support. I, too, remained connected, serving as a national council member for ACS's childhood cancer initiative, Gold Together for Childhood Cancer.

Our paths crossed again, as paths often do when they are guided by shared purpose. Tony's passion for helping cancer patients is not expressed merely in words. It is proven through action. Again and again, he chooses to show up for others. It blesses my heart to witness all that he continues to accomplish, knowing how deeply leukemia shaped his early life. He could have easily walked away from the world of cancer, closing that chapter forever once survival was secured.

But Tony chose differently. He walks into that darkness every day, to be a voice for children who are still fighting, to stand beside families who are afraid, and to shine hope in places that often feel cruel and unforgiving. His life is a testament to the truth that survival is not just about living. It is about what you do with the life you were given. This book is proof of that.

Tony Garcia

# Chapter 1
## *The Summer My Life Changed Forever*

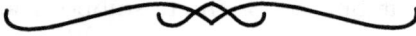

$It$ began on a warm summer day in Texas, August 14, 1973, when the heat lay thick and unmoving, as if the air itself had decided to take a long rest. I was only two and a half years old, too young to understand the world or remember its details clearly, yet old enough to feel the things that mattered most. Love, laughter, and the steady comfort of home.

Our house was filled with the goodness of ordinary life. Sunshine peeked through the windows. Birds chirped their endless songs. Somewhere, a fan turned lazily, pushing warm air from one room to the next. My parents moved through the day as they always did, unaware that time was quietly splitting itself into a before and after.

That afternoon, the first signs of terror arrived. A small cough. A warm forehead. Nothing alarming, just the kind of thing that normally happened to children in summer. My mom noticed I wasn't quite myself. I was quieter, clung to her leg longer than usual, and rested my head against her shoulder instead of running off to play. She pressed her lips to my forehead and frowned slightly.

"It's probably the heat," she said, more to herself than to anyone else.

"Or maybe he's just worn out."

By evening, the fever lingered. My mom gave me medicine, tucked me into bed, and stayed close, listening to my breathing long after the house had gone quiet. By morning, the fever hadn't broken. Instead, it burned brighter, stubborn and unyielding. I moved slowly now, my small body heavy, as if gravity itself had changed overnight.

The next day passed in a blur of worry and watchfulness. My mom checked my temperature repeatedly. She wiped my forehead with a cool cloth. My dad came home early from work, his voice low and concerned as he asked the same question everyone asks in moments like these, "Is he any better?"

I was not.

Two days later, on August 16, my mom wrapped me in her arms and carried me into our local pediatrician's office. The waiting room smelled faintly of antiseptic and crayons. Plastic chairs lined the walls. A few other children sat quietly, their parents flipping through worn magazines. I was limp against my mom's chest, my head resting in the hollow of her shoulder.

The doctor examined me carefully. She checked my ears, pressed gently on my neck, and peered into my throat. She smiled kindly, the way doctors do when they want to reassure more than diagnose.

"It's tonsillitis," she said. "Nothing unusual."

She gave me a shot of penicillin and told my mom I'd be fine in a few days. "Children bounce back quickly," she said. My mom nodded, relief and doubt warring quietly inside her. My dad wanted to believe it, too. They both did. Parents cling to hope when it is offered, especially when it comes wrapped in authority. We went home.

But I wasn't fine.

The days that followed were slow and uneasy. Instead of improving, I began to slip away in small, almost imperceptible ways. My laughter, once easy and frequent, grew rare. My appetite faded. Toys lay untouched where they had once been scattered joyfully across the floor. I slept more, stirred less, and when I did wake, my eyes no longer sparkled the way they had before.

My mom noticed everything.

She later said she could see it in my skin first, that strange, unnatural paleness that did not belong to a sun-kissed Texas toddler. She said I looked "washed out," as if the color had been gently drained from me, leaving something fragile behind. She studied my face in the soft light of the house, searching for the child she knew so well.

Each night, she lay awake listening to me breathe.

Two weeks passed like this. Two long weeks of quiet fear, unanswered questions, and the growing sense that something was terribly wrong. Still, nothing prepared them for August 31.

That day, I fell and hit my lower lip. It was a small tumble, the kind children take every day. Nothing dramatic. No sharp cry. Just a startled gasp and a bit of blood. My mom scooped me up instinctively, murmuring comfort as she pressed a cloth to my mouth.

But the bleeding didn't stop.

Minutes passed. The cloth soaked through. My parents exchanged worried glances as they tried to slow the flow. Blood continued to spill, far more than it should have for such a minor injury. Panic crept in quietly at first, then all at once. Eventually, the bleeding slowed and stopped, but the unease remained, heavy and unshakable.

That night, my parents barely slept.

The next morning, September 1, I woke up feverish again. My skin was pale, almost translucent. I didn't cry. I didn't ask to be held. I didn't ask for anything at all. I simply lay there, still and quiet, my small body exhausted by a fight no one yet understood.

I didn't want to play. I didn't want to eat. I barely moved.

My mom said it felt like watching me disappear in front of her eyes.

She sat beside my bed, brushing my hair back again and again, whispering my name as if saying it might anchor me to the world. From September 1 through September 3, I barely left that bed. The house grew unnaturally quiet, as if it, too, was holding its breath.

Every night, my parents prayed. They prayed in whispers so I wouldn't hear the fear in their voices. They prayed for answers, for healing, for time. They prayed that whatever this was would pass, that the next morning would bring relief, that the doctor had been right.

But it didn't pass.

And by the third night, they knew. Deep down, in that place where truth settles before words, that this was only the beginning.

# Chapter 2
## *The Diagnosis That Changed Everything*

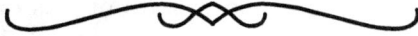

$\mathcal{O}$n September 6, 1973, my pediatrician finally ordered a blood culture. By then, worry had become a constant presence in our home, no longer something that came and went but something that settled into the walls and followed my parents from room to room. The test results came back the next day, negative for beta-strep. No infection. No simple explanation. My parents were told to bring me back in for more tests.

Something was definitely wrong. We could all feel it, even though we had no idea how wrong it was.

By Friday, September 7, I was admitted to our local hospital. At two and a half years old, I was far too young to understand what hospitals meant, but I could feel the fear. The smells were sharp and unfamiliar. The lights were too bright. Strange hands touched me, lifted me, restrained me. My pediatrician ordered a blood transfusion, but when the nurses tried to start an IV, they couldn't find a vein. My veins had collapsed.

They tried again. And again. Each attempt ended the same way. Another failure, another quiet exchange between nurses, another glance toward my parents that said more than words could. Eventually, one of them made a small incision on my left ankle to draw blood directly. It was a horrible solution, but there were no other options left. The cut was painful, and it left a scar I still carry today, a visible reminder that has followed me through life, a mark from the moment my body began to betray me.

That evening, the bloodwork came back with results no one wanted to see. My white blood cell count was dangerously high, so high it could not be explained away. My pediatrician, who had known me since infancy, began to suspect leukemia. The word itself hung in the air, heavy and unfamiliar.

Leukemia is a cancer of the blood-forming tissues, mainly the bone marrow. Normally, marrow makes red blood cells that carry oxygen, white blood cells that fight infection, and platelets that help the blood to clot. In leukemia, abnormal white blood cells grow uncontrollably, crowding out healthy cells and weakening the body.

Leukemia is a group of related cancers, classified by speed and cell type. Acute leukemias progress quickly and need immediate treatment, while chronic leukemias grow slowly and may be monitored before therapy.

Leukemias also depend on cell origin: lymphocytic leukemias come from immune cells, and myeloid leukemias from cells that make red blood cells, platelets, and some white blood cells.

This creates four main types: Acute Lymphoblastic Leukemia (ALL), the most common in children; Acute Myeloid Leukemia (AML), which affects children and adults; Chronic Lymphocytic Leukemia (CLL), which usually occurs in older adults; and Chronic Myeloid Leukemia (CML), which is linked to the Philadelphia chromosome. There are also rarer subtypes, showing how complex blood cancers can be.

The next morning, September 8, 1973, I was taken for a bone marrow biopsy. A bone marrow biopsy is a procedure used to examine the soft, spongy tissue inside bones where blood cells are made, often to diagnose or monitor diseases such as leukemia. In that era, especially for children, this procedure was far more traumatic than it is today. Sedation was limited or unavailable in many hospitals, and pain management options were minimal. Young patients were often awake and physically restrained while a large needle was inserted into the hip bone to extract marrow, a process that could be frightening and painful. Emotional preparation and child-centered care were rarely part of the experience, and parents were often kept at a distance.

Modern bone marrow biopsies are typically performed with a strong emphasis on comfort, dignity, and emotional well-being. Children today often receive sedation or general anesthesia, along with local numbing agents, so they feel little to no pain. Child life specialists help explain the procedure in age-appropriate ways, reduce fear, and provide coping tools. Parents are encouraged to be present, and the entire process is designed to be as gentle and quick as possible. While the procedure itself remains medically similar, the experience has been transformed, shifting from something endured in fear to one guided by compassion, safety, and respect for the child's emotional needs.

Because I was only a toddler, I was sedated for my biopsy. For my parents, it meant handing their baby over to strangers yet again into cold rooms filled with machines, needles, and procedures they did not understand but were forced to trust. Fear left no space for questions. There was no choice, no pause, no time to breathe, only the terrifying necessity of letting go.

I remember fragments of that day, not full scenes, but sensations and flashes that have stayed with me in ways memory often does when trauma arrives before language is fully formed. I remember the coldness of the room. I remember being held down. I remember pain, sharp and confusing, arriving without explanation.

And I remember believing, deeply and sincerely, that I was being punished.

At two and a half years old, I didn't understand illness or disease. I understood rules. I understood being good and being bad. And so, in my young mind, pain being inflicted upon me meant I had done something wrong. I remember crying out, "I'll be good, I promise!" as if that might make it stop. I remember my parents crying too, their faces distorted by fear and helplessness, my mom gripping my hand and telling me over and over that I hadn't done anything wrong. That I was brave. That I was loved.

Those words mattered. They still do.

That night, my parents sat in a quiet hospital room, surrounded by equipment and uncertainty, trying to make sense of a world they had never imagined entering. They were suddenly being asked to consider treatments, probabilities, and decisions no parent should have to make, especially not for a toddler who couldn't even understand what was happening to him.

When my pediatrician came into the room, she was crying. Doctors aren't supposed to cry. At least, that's what people believe. But she did. And in that moment, my parents knew before she spoke that their lives had already changed.

**"Your son has acute lymphocytic leukemia,"** she said.

Those words shattered everything.

In 1973, childhood leukemia was almost always a death sentence. Survival rates hovered somewhere between ten and twenty percent, depending on the study, depending on the hospital, depending on how much hope one was willing to allow. There were no reassuring statistics. No long-term survivor stories to cling to. There was only uncertainty and fear.

But my parents refused to accept that this was the end of my story.

The very next day, September 9, I was referred to MD Anderson Cancer Center in Houston, Texas, one of the few places in the country actively pioneering treatments for children like me. Their first choice had been St. Jude Children's Research Hospital in Memphis, Tennessee. Even then, St. Jude represented the gold standard of pediatric cancer care. But it was out of reach, both financially and geographically. The distance alone meant long journeys, missed work, and expenses they simply could not manage.

Reality narrowed their options quickly.

And so, Houston became our destination.

Looking back now, with decades of hindsight, I understand how close I came to not surviving, not because of the disease alone, but because of circumstance, timing, and access. I understand how fragile the line was between life and death, how dependent survival was on geography, money, and the emerging edge of medical science.

At the time, though, I was just a small toddler being carried from one place to another, unaware that my life had already become a series of decisions made by frightened adults who loved me fiercely.

Leukemia entered my life before I could pronounce the word, before I could spell my name, before I could understand what survival meant. It arrived quietly, without warning, and it would shape everything that followed.

This was the first step into a fight that would change us forever.

# Chapter 3
*The Long Road to Survival*

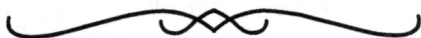

In Houston, the fight for my life truly began. The University of Texas MD Anderson Cancer Center lies in the heart of the famous Texas Medical Center. To understand the magnitude of an institution like MD Anderson and its significance in the war on cancer, it is important to understand its history.

MD Anderson did not begin as a grand idea. It began the way most lasting things do, with quiet resolve, careful stewardship, and a refusal to accept limits.

The man whose name the hospital bears, Monroe Dunaway Anderson, was not a physician. He was a businessman shaped by the post-Civil War South, raised on thrift, discipline, and responsibility. He made his fortune through patience, building what would become one of the largest cotton trading companies in the world. Wealth, to him, was not something to display. It was something to put to work.

When he created the foundation that would later fund

MD Anderson Cancer Center, he did not dictate how it must be used. He trusted others to decide wisely. After his death in 1939, the trustees recognized an opportunity that few at the time fully understood: **cancer was becoming one of the great battles of modern medicine**, and Texas needed a place devoted entirely to fighting it.

In 1941, the Texas Legislature authorized the creation of a state cancer hospital. It was an idea without a home, without certainty, and without adequate funding. The MD Anderson Foundation stepped in, agreeing to match the state's appropriation on one condition: that the hospital be built in Houston and bear Monroe Anderson's name. It was a practical decision, but also a visionary one. Houston would become the center of a medical experiment whose consequences would ripple far beyond Texas.

The hospital's earliest days were modest, even improvised. During World War II, construction materials were scarce, doctors were deployed overseas, and priorities lay elsewhere. MD Anderson began operating out of temporary quarters, treating a handful of patients in buildings never meant for medicine. But even then, something important was happening. Cancer was being studied not as a side concern, but as the central mission.

Soon, MD Anderson grew deliberately, guided by a belief that treatment and research belonged together. Patients were not just cases to be managed, but were part of a larger effort to understand a disease that medicine had barely begun to confront.

By the time I arrived there in 1973, MD Anderson had already earned a reputation as one of the few places in the country willing to take on childhood leukemia with seriousness and urgency. This was not a hospital offering comfort alone. It was a hospital willing to push boundaries, to try treatments that were still being refined, to accept uncertainty in exchange for the possibility of survival. That mattered.

When my parents brought me to Houston, they were not choosing a miracle. They were choosing the best chance available in a world where guarantees did not exist. MD Anderson represented effort, rigor, and hope grounded in work, not promises.

I did not know any of this then. I was too young to understand legacies or foundations or the long arc of medical progress. But my life unfolded inside the walls built by those decisions. The treatments that saved me were possible only because a man decades earlier had believed wealth carried responsibility, and because a group of physicians believed cancer deserved singular focus.

MD Anderson was not just where I was treated. It was where survival was being invented.

By the time we arrived in Houston, my parents had already crossed an invisible threshold, leaving behind the comfort of familiarity and stepping into a world ruled by protocols, probabilities, and machines.

MD Anderson was not just a hospital. It was a place where hope and fear lived side by side, where children like me were being treated with therapies that were still, in many ways, experimental.

In the early 1970s, there were no settled roadmaps for childhood leukemia. Protocols were being written as they were being lived. The drugs flowing into my veins had been tested in laboratories and in small trials, but not yet across generations of survivors. Dosages were adjusted by observation. Side effects were documented in real time. What worked for one child might fail for the next, and no one could say with certainty why.

In that sense, we were not just patients. We were evidence. Each child in those wards represented a question medicine had not yet answered. *Would this combination of drugs stop the disease? Would the damage be temporary or permanent? Could a young body endure what was required to save it?* The answers were not found in textbooks. They were learned at the bedside, over months and years, through outcomes that were sometimes hopeful and sometimes devastating.

I did not sign consent forms, but I lived inside their consequences. For us kids with leukemia, our parents agreed to treatments that carried no guarantees, guided by doctors who spoke honestly about uncertainty. There was no illusion of safety, only the faint promise of possibility. Choosing treatment meant choosing risk, not as an abstract idea, but as something that could alter a child forever, even in survival.

Looking back now, it would be easy to call us guinea pigs. In a literal sense, we were. Our bodies absorbed therapies still being refined, our responses recorded and studied so that others might one day fare better. But that word alone does not capture the full truth. We were not experimented on out of carelessness or ambition. We were fought for!

Those doctors stood at the edge of what medicine knew and stepped forward anyway, carrying our parents' trust with them. Every gain came at a cost, paid in side effects, long hospital stays, and lives permanently changed. Progress was not clean. It was earned through children who endured more than they should have had to.

I survived because of that imperfect process. Because someone before me had survived just long enough to teach doctors what to try next. And the children who came after me would have better odds than I did.

Hope and fear shared the same rooms in the pediatric cancer clinic. They sat together in waiting areas, walked the same hallways, and stood quietly at bedsides. Survival was never promised. It was negotiated carefully, painfully, one child at a time.

On September 12, 1973, I began chemotherapy. The drugs Vincristine, prednisone, methotrexate, hydrocortisone, Adriamycin, and Cytoxan were part of a regimen that was still being developed and refined. Doctors were learning in real time how much the human body could endure, especially the body of a child. These medications were powerful, aggressive, and unforgiving. They were designed to kill cancer, but they did not distinguish carefully between what was sick and what was healthy.

Almost immediately, my body began to change. My hair fell out in soft clumps, leaving my scalp bare and sensitive. My appetite disappeared, replaced by nausea and fatigue. My small frame weakened, my limbs thin and unsteady. I grew quiet, conserving energy without understanding why. I did not know the names of the drugs flowing into my veins, nor could I understand the danger they were meant to counter. All I knew was that something relentless had taken hold of my life. And yet, even then, something else was forming.

I did not recognize it at the time, but my spirit was being tempered, shaped under pressure like steel. Strength, I would later learn, does not always announce itself. Sometimes it grows silently, forged in places where choice has been taken away.

On October 16, 1973, the fight escalated. I underwent radiation therapy to my skull, a preventative measure meant to keep the leukemia from spreading to my brain. The procedure itself was frightening, even for an adult. For a child, it was incomprehensible. I was immobilized, positioned with precision, surrounded by machines that roared with menace. My parents watched, in helpless horror, trusting that the damage being done was necessary, hopeful it was not permanent.

The radiation did its job. The cancer was held at bay. But it left invisible scars. Moderately severe post-radiation changes in my central nervous system would follow me for the rest of my life.

As I grew, those changes revealed themselves in ways no one could have predicted at the time. The damage was not dramatic or immediately obvious. It did not announce itself all at once. Instead, it appeared slowly, in classrooms and at kitchen tables, in the quiet frustration of trying to keep up. Learning challenges took shape where confidence should have been forming. My thinking was a bit slower. There were moments when I understood the classroom material but couldn't reach it quickly enough, when the answer felt just out of grasp, trapped behind a delay I couldn't explain.

School was simply much harder for me than it was for others. Reading took longer, not because I couldn't read, but because comprehension arrived in pieces rather than all at once. I reread pages while classmates moved on. Instructions had to be heard twice, sometimes three times, before they settled. Processing information required more effort, more patience, and more energy than anyone could see. By the time I had finished one task, others were already starting the next.

What made it hardest was that my determination never lagged behind my ability. I wanted to succeed. I studied longer, tried harder, pushed myself further, often without the results to show for it. Teachers sometimes mistook that gap for a lack of effort. Peers mistook it for a lack of intelligence. I learned early how quietly a child can feel diminished without anyone intending to do harm.

Over time, I adapted. I learned to compensate where I could, to work around what would not change. Persistence became a skill as important as reading or math. I discovered that understanding might come slowly, but once it arrived, it stayed. The lessons I learned were durable, earned through repetition and refusal to quit. I refused to be defined by what had been taken from me.

With the unwavering support of my family, teachers who believed in me, and friends who never saw me as less than capable, I found ways to adapt. I learned persistence before I learned multiplication. I learned resilience before I learned grammar. I graduated from elementary school. Then high school. And eventually, against odds that had once seemed insurmountable, I earned a college degree. Each milestone was not just an achievement. It was a quiet act of defiance.

From 1973 through 1983, my life followed a routine that few children know. Hospitals replaced playgrounds. Needles replaced toys. Hospital stays stretched on for weeks, sometimes months, punctuated by brief returns home that never lasted long enough. Bone marrow biopsies. Spinal taps. Hair loss that came and went. An endless cycle of hope followed by fear, relief followed by uncertainty. Just when life began to feel normal again, we were pulled back into the sterile world of oncology wards and waiting rooms.

Through it all, my mom never left my side. She became my constant, my anchor in a world that rarely made sense. She made sure I ate balanced meals every day, even when my appetite was gone, and the food tasted wrong. She ensured I took my medicine on time, insisted on vegetables, and believed fiercely in the role nutrition played in survival. She was right. Many children didn't make it, not only because of the disease, but also because their bodies were too weak to endure the treatment.

My mom fought alongside me every single day. She was my advocate when I could not speak for myself. My protector when fear threatened to overwhelm. My source of strength when my own ran thin. Without her vigilance, her resolve, and her refusal to give in to despair, I would not be here today.

My dad carried his pain differently. He was strong but tender, steady in ways that mattered most. He bore his heartbreak quietly, providing stability when everything else felt uncertain. My siblings, two older sisters and an older brother, learned early what courage looked like, what love demanded, and how a family can bend without breaking.

Many people are unaware of just how profoundly childhood cancer impacts an entire family, not just the child who is diagnosed. Almost immediately, families are forced into survival mode. Parents often have to divide responsibilities and physically separate, with one becoming a full-time caregiver at hospitals and appointments while the other works multiple jobs to cover mounting medical bills and keep food on the table.

Siblings are frequently shuffled between relatives, friends, or caregivers, their routines and sense of stability disrupted as the family struggles to cope.

What makes this even more devastating is that childhood cancer is rarely a short-term crisis. Treatments, setbacks, and uncertainty can stretch on for months or even years, placing relentless emotional, financial, and physical strain on everyone involved. Families can become fractured under the weight of it all, not from lack of love, but from exhaustion and survival. The toll of childhood cancer is deep, lasting, and truly heartbreaking.

Cancer took ten years of my childhood. It took time that can never be reclaimed. Years of innocence were replaced by hospital rooms, treatments, and fear. It took from my family as well, reshaping our lives around survival, dividing our attention, our energy, and often our sense of normalcy. We measured time in appointments and outcomes, learned to live with uncertainty, and carried a weight that never truly lifted.

But cancer gave me something, too. It gave me a lifelong understanding of endurance, a deep gratitude for ordinary moments, and an awareness of the quiet, unwavering strength of the people who stand beside us when survival is the only goal. Those years shaped who I became, teaching me that even in what is taken, something lasting can still be forged.

Tony Garcia

# Chapter 4
## *The Relapses*

*O*n April 22, 1976, when I was just five years old, my right testicle swelled. By then, my parents knew better than to dismiss anything unusual. Childhood leukemia had already taught them caution. Tests followed quickly. A biopsy confirmed what everyone feared, but no one wanted to say aloud: leukemic infiltration. The cancer had returned.

Relapse is a word that sounds clinical and contained. In reality, it is an earthquake. I underwent radiation therapy to both testicles almost immediately. There was no time for deliberation, no opportunity to weigh distant consequences against immediate need. The goal was survival. The cost, though not fully understood at the time, was permanent. The radiation destroyed my ability to father children later in life. It was a loss I would not comprehend until adulthood, when the idea of legacy, family, and continuation finally came into focus.

At five years old, I only knew that the treatments were harsher this time. My body, already marked by years of chemotherapy and radiation, responded with greater resistance. Fatigue deepened. My skin burned and peeled. Pain became more familiar than comfort. I learned early that survival was not a single event, but a process, one that demanded repeated sacrifices.

This is the part of childhood cancer most people never see. Treatment does not end when the cancer retreats. It leaves behind a landscape altered in ways that unfold slowly over years and decades. For children like me, the body becomes a place of negotiations between what was saved and what was lost, between resilience and damage that cannot be undone.

By the time I reached school age, side effects were no longer temporary visitors. They were companions. Hormonal disruption. Delayed growth. Cognitive challenges made learning slower and more exhausting. My immune system remained fragile, forcing constant vigilance against infections that others shrugged off. Doctors monitored my development carefully, measuring not just height and weight, but what had been compromised beneath the surface.

Even then, the full extent of the long-term and late effects was still unknown. Pediatric oncology in the 1970s was focused, understandably, on survival. Little was known about what happened decades later to children whose bodies were exposed to chemotherapy and radiation at such an early age. The question was not "how will this child live?" but "will this child live at all?" I was still alive. That was the victory.

Then came October 10, 1980. I was nine years old when I suffered a bone marrow relapse. Of all the moments in my childhood, that day stands apart with a clarity that time has never softened. I remember the exam room at MD Anderson. I remember the way the air felt heavier, the way my doctor's voice changed before the words were spoken. I remember watching my mom's face as she absorbed the news that the cancer had returned, deeper this time, more dangerous. We cried together.

I wrapped my arms around her and held on as tightly as I could, as if physical closeness might protect us both from what lay ahead. Then she did something extraordinary. She told me that the decision to continue treatment was mine. That even though I was just a boy, I had the right to choose. Most children are not asked to make such decisions. Our bodies do not seem to belong to us. We do not get to choose what we eat, what we wear, when we get poked or prodded, or what nasty drugs are pumped into our tiny veins. We are just forced to comply. Yet here I was being given permission to choose what happened to my own body.

I understood more than people might expect. I understood pain. I understood hospitals. I understood what it meant to be tired in a way sleep could not fix. I also understood that stopping meant dying. The choice, though framed as freedom, was stark.

I looked at my mom through tears and told her I wanted to fight. I wasn't ready to go. That day, I made the first conscious decision of my life. I decided to survive.

The treatments that followed were among the most aggressive I would endure. More chemotherapy. More hospitalizations. More invasive procedures. Bone marrow biopsies became routine. Spinal taps punctuated my childhood. My body endured cumulative damage that would remain long after remission was achieved.

As an adult, I now understand what my younger self could not, that surviving childhood cancer often means living with its aftermath. Late effects emerge quietly. Cardiac issues, endocrine dysfunction, infertility, cognitive impairment, and increased risk of secondary cancers. Survivorship is not a clean ending. It is a lifelong condition. And yet, I survived. Not untouched, not unchanged, but alive.

The child who chose to fight could not imagine the man he would become, carrying both the scars and the strength forged in those years. That choice did not make me fearless. It made me endure. It taught me that life is not defined by what is taken from us, but by what we decide to do with what remains. I chose to stay. And that choice shaped everything that followed.

# Chapter 5

*The End of Treatment*

On October 4, 1983, when I was twelve years old, after ten long years of treatment at MD Anderson, my doctor finally said the words I had dreamed of hearing, words that felt almost too impossible to believe: "No more chemotherapy."

For a moment, the world seemed to stop. In that exam room, the fluorescent lights shone brightly overhead, and the air smelled like antiseptic and something faintly metallic, a scent that had become as familiar to me as my own skin. I was cancer–free! Those words sounded triumphant, celebratory, explosive.

I don't remember everything the doctor said after that. I'm sure there were explanations, cautions, follow-ups, and medical language carefully chosen to temper hope with realism. But all of it faded into the background, muffled and distant. What I remember most clearly is my mom's soft and trembling voice, barely more than a whisper, as she said, "Thank you, Lord." It wasn't just gratitude. It was surrender.

For ten years, my mom had lived in a constant state of prayer. She prayed in hospital rooms while machines beeped and bags full of poison pumped into her little boy's body. She prayed in church pews, gripping the wood in front of her as if it were the only thing keeping her upright. She prayed beside my bed at night, long after I had fallen asleep, tracing the outline of my small body with her eyes, memorizing every breath as if afraid God might ask her to give me back. She prayed when doctors spoke honestly and when they spoke gently. She prayed when hope was strong and when it felt completely impossible.

Now, in that moment, her prayers had been answered. I was old enough to understand what a victory this was, and old enough to know it wasn't the kind of victory people imagine. There were no balloons tied to my wrist, no confetti falling from the ceiling. Cancer didn't leave politely or cleanly. It left marks. It left open wounds. It left a body and a mind that had been shaped by years of poison meant to save it. Even as a twelve-year-old, I understood something important. The healing was not complete.

The treatments had done what they were designed to do. They had kept me alive. But they had also taken their toll. Cognitive challenges lingered, subtle but persistent, like shadows I couldn't step away from no matter how bright the light became. My body carried scars, some visible, some hidden, that reminded me every day of what it had endured. And infertility, a word far too heavy for a child, settled quietly into my future, altering dreams I didn't yet know how to articulate.

These weren't footnotes to my survival. They were chapters of it. There were moments when those reminders felt unfair. I had survived something most children never face, yet survival came with a cost that followed me long after the hospital doors closed behind us. I would later learn that this is the truth for so many childhood cancer survivors. The disease may be gone, but the consequences remain. Long-term effects are health challenges that begin during cancer treatment and continue after treatment has ended. These effects may require ongoing monitoring or care as a child grows and can affect daily life well beyond the active treatment phase. Late effects are health issues that do not appear right away but develop months or even years after cancer treatment has finished. Because a child's body and brain are still developing, these effects can emerge over time and may change as the survivor reaches adolescence and adulthood. All of these are invisible battles that don't end when the treatment does.

But even then, standing on the threshold between sickness and something resembling normal life, I sensed that these reminders were not my defeat. They became my teachers.

They taught me endurance, not the dramatic kind celebrated in stories, but the quiet, daily kind that shows up even when you're tired of being strong. They taught me patience, especially with myself, on days when my mind moved slower or my body reminded me of its limits. They taught me compassion because once you have suffered deeply, you recognize pain in others even when they try to hide it. Most of all, they taught me that nothing is guaranteed.

Every breath is a gift. Every sunrise is undeserved grace. Every tomorrow is something to be received with humility, not entitlement. While other children took health for granted, I learned early that life is fragile and, therefore, sacred.

Looking back now, I can see what I could not fully understand then. My mom's faith carried us through when strength alone would not have been enough. There were days when strength ran out. Days when answers didn't come. Days when the future looked terrifyingly uncertain. Faith stepped in where human endurance failed.

My mom's prayers were not loud or showy. They were whispered in the dark when no one else could hear. They were spoken through tears when words felt inadequate. They were sometimes nothing more than a plea. "Please. Just please. Let him live."

Those prayers were answered, but not all at once, and not without cost. They were answered in time, in process, in survival shaped by sacrifice. God did not erase the journey. He walked us through it.

That day, October 4, 1983, was more than the end of my treatment. It was a marker in my life, a dividing line between who I had been and who I was becoming. It was proof that faith can carry you through the fire and bring you out refined, not destroyed. Scarred, yes. Changed forever, absolutely. But still here.

My parents believed that God had spared me for a reason. They didn't know what that reason was, and they didn't pretend to. They simply trusted that my life had purpose beyond survival. It would take me many years, years of struggle, growth, doubt, and reflection, to begin to understand what that might mean.

But even now, I believe it too. I was not saved just to exist. I was saved to live. To bear witness. To carry the story of survival, faith, and perseverance forward. Cancer took much from me, but it did not take my life, and it did not take my ability to find meaning in the pain.

On that day, when the words "No more chemotherapy" finally came true, something else was born alongside my freedom. A responsibility to honor the life I was given. And every day since has been my answer to that gift.

Tony Garcia

# Chapter 6
*The Man Who Lived*

As I grew older, I began to understand just how extraordinary my survival truly was. As a child, I knew only that I was sick, that hospitals felt like a second home, and that needles, masks, and whispered conversations followed me everywhere. I did not yet understand statistics or odds. I did not know that in the 1970s, children like me were rarely expected to live.

Acute lymphocytic leukemia was not something doctors spoke of with confidence or hope. It was a quiet, devastating sentence, delivered with lowered voices and guarded expressions. Survival was the exception. In fact, not long before, 100% of children with leukemia died. They literally bled to death on gurneys in hospitals around the nation and the world within a month of their diagnosis. When chemotherapy was first used in children, people (including doctors) thought it too cruel to attempt. Obviously, there is some validity to this, as those treatments often would kill the kids even if the cancer did not. Yet, there I was. Alive. I had beaten the odds.

That truth didn't fully sink in until years later, when I was old enough to look back and realize just how narrow that path had been. I was one of the few children who made it through a disease that claimed so many others. I carried their absence with me, even before I had the words for grief or survivor's guilt. I had been given something precious: time. And I didn't yet know what to do with it.

As a teenager, the cost of survival began to reveal itself in quieter, more complicated ways. The treatments that saved my life had left their mark. Radiation had touched my brain, chemotherapy had pushed my body far beyond what it was ever meant to endure, and the effects followed me into the classroom. I struggled to keep up. Learning felt slow and uneven, like trying to run through water while everyone else moved freely on land. Words sometimes slipped through my grasp. Numbers blurred. Focus came and went without warning. There were days when my mind felt wrapped in fog, and no matter how hard I tried, I couldn't push through it.

School wasn't easy, and neither was the way I saw myself within it. I was aware that I wasn't like the other kids. What they absorbed effortlessly took everything I had. Teachers tried to help, but not everyone understood. Back then, we didn't talk much about cognitive late effects or treatment-related challenges. I often felt alone, frustrated, and embarrassed, wondering why survival hadn't come with a clean slate. But giving up was never an option.

Somewhere inside me lived the promise I had made as a nine-year-old boy, a promise made in fear and pain, but rooted in determination. I had decided that if I was going to live, I was going to fight for that life. I carried that promise into every classroom, every test, every setback. When my confidence faltered, my parents carried it for me, reminding me that surviving wasn't just about staying alive. Survival meant effort. It meant trying when quitting would have been easier. It meant showing up even when the outcome was uncertain.

My mom believed in that truth fiercely. She reminded me, again and again, that persistence mattered more than speed, and courage mattered more than perfection. My dad showed me, through his steady work and quiet sacrifice, what endurance looked like. Together, they taught me that survival wasn't passive. It was active, ongoing, and deeply human.

The physical scars eventually faded. The marks on my body softened into pale reminders of battles already fought. But the emotional scars lingered. For years, fear followed me like a shadow. Every check-up reopened old wounds. Every unexplained fever sent my heart racing. I learned to live with vigilance, always listening to my body, always waiting for the other shoe to drop. Cancer doesn't simply leave when the treatment ends. It stays with you, in your thoughts, your memories, your instincts.

Even as an adult, I carried that awareness. I understood that you don't walk away from something like leukemia. You live alongside it. You adapt. You learn how to breathe again without forgetting what it felt like to nearly stop breathing at all. Over time, I made peace with that truth.

There were other losses I had to face as I grew older, losses that weren't immediately visible. I learned that I couldn't father children, a reality I hadn't fully grasped until adulthood. The knowledge hit hard. It was painful to realize that the medicine that saved my life had also taken away the possibility of creating life. I mourned what could never be, and I allowed myself to feel that grief fully.

But grief, like survival, evolves. Slowly, I came to understand that nurturing life takes many forms. It lives in mentorship, in compassion, in the way we show up for others. It lives in listening, in encouraging, in offering kindness when the world feels heavy. I learned that legacy isn't always written in blood. It's written in love.

In August of 1989, I began testosterone therapy to replace what radiation had stolen from my body. That chapter marked another step in my long recovery. The therapy helped restore balance, strength, and stability, physical reminders that healing doesn't happen all at once. Recovery isn't a moment. It's a lifetime of adjustments, acceptance, and renewal. Each step forward mattered, no matter how small.

Now, when I look in the mirror, I don't see just a survivor. I see a man shaped by endurance. I see the faint line on my left ankle from that first transfusion attempt. I see invisible scars left by radiation and chemotherapy. I see determination in my eyes, a gentle but unshakable reminder that I made it through something that should have taken me.

Every breath I take feels borrowed, not in fear, but in gratitude. Survival wasn't just a product of medicine or chance. It was love. It was a mom who refused to leave my side. A dad who worked tirelessly to hold our family together. Doctors and nurses who fought alongside me. And a God who carried me when my strength was gone.

I have learned that life after cancer isn't about pretending the pain never existed. It's about honoring the truth that you were forever changed and choosing to let that change give your life meaning. I am the boy who almost died. But I am also the man who lived.

And every day, I choose to live fully, not just for myself, but for every child who fought, every child who survived, and every child who didn't get the chance to grow older and tell their story.

Tony Garcia

# Chapter 7

## *The Purpose*

$\mathcal{I}$ did not write this story to relieve the pain. I wrote it to remember the purpose.

Pain has never needed reminding. It has a way of returning on its own, uninvited, unexpected, and unrelenting. Pain lives in the body, in memory, in moments that catch us off guard when we least expect it. Writing this book did not erase what happened to me, nor did it soften every hard memory. If anything, it brought many of them into sharper focus. But this story was never about escaping pain. It was about understanding why I lived through it.

For most of my life, the story of my illness existed quietly within my family. It was spoken of in fragments, in hushed conversations, in knowing looks exchanged across a room. It was a miracle we protected, not because we were ashamed, but because it was sacred. It carried gratitude so deep it was almost unbearable, and grief so heavy it sometimes went unspoken. We learned to hold both at the same time.

As a child, I didn't understand the weight of what I had survived. I only knew that something terrible had happened, and somehow, it ended with me still here. As I grew older, that awareness matured. I began to understand that survival wasn't just a medical outcome or a fortunate statistic. It was a responsibility. It asked something of me. It asked whether I would let the miracle end with me, or whether I would allow it to ripple outward into something greater.

This memoir exists because I came to believe that survival is not meant to be silent. Stories matter. They carry truth in a way facts cannot. They move where explanations fail. They remind us that pain has context, that suffering is shared, and that even the most isolating experiences are never entirely ours alone. I believe that stories have the power to heal, not because they fix what is broken, but because they name it. Because they say, "I see you. I've been there. You are not imagining the weight you carry."

Somewhere, as these words are read, a parent is sitting beside a hospital bed. The room is too quiet, broken only by the steady hum of machines and the soft rise and fall of a child's chest. That parent is whispering prayers into the dark, bargaining with God, hoping for just one more day, one more chance, one more miracle. Somewhere else, a child is fighting a battle they cannot yet understand, enduring pain they don't have words for, trusting adults they barely know, being brave simply because they have no other choice.

To them, I want this story to say, "Miracles do not always arrive quickly. They do not always look the way we expect. Sometimes they come wrapped in scars, setbacks, and years of unanswered questions. Sometimes they come quietly, after the storm has passed, when survival itself feels almost unbelievable. But they do come. And when they do, they change us forever.

Writing my story felt like walking back through time. Each chapter carried me to places I hadn't visited in years. Hospital hallways, childhood bedrooms, moments of fear and faith that shaped who I would become. I revisited faces I loved, some still with me, others only in memory. I felt again the vulnerability of a body that couldn't protect itself and the fierce love of people who refused to let me face it alone.

This journey reminded me how fragile life truly is. How easily it can be altered, interrupted, or taken away. But it also reminded me of something equally powerful. Love is stronger than fragility. Love shows up when answers are scarce. Love sits in uncomfortable rooms and stays long after hope fades. Love holds vigil in the dark and believes in a fresh new morning even when the night feels endless.

My parents taught me that lesson long before I could name it. They showed me that hope is not denial. It is defiance. Hope does not ignore pain or pretend suffering isn't real. Hope looks directly at the worst possible outcome and says, "I will still believe in tomorrow." Hope is the courage to keep loving, keep fighting, keep praying, even when your heart feels like it might break.

I wrote this book to honor them, my parents, who are no longer here, but whose love remains woven into every page of my life. My mom never left my side, not for a moment, not when the nights were long or the outcomes uncertain. She was my constant in a world that felt like it was unraveling. When fear tried to take hold, she stood firm, carrying strength I did not yet have, and faith I could not yet fully understand. She fought for me with a quiet ferocity, challenging despair with prayer, exhaustion with resolve, and doubt with unwavering love. She was a warrior in every sense of the word, standing watch over her child when the battle seemed impossible to win.

My dad fought differently, but no less fiercely. He carried his pain in silence, shouldering responsibility so the rest of us could keep going. He worked, he prayed, and he endured, even as his own heart was breaking. He took on multiple jobs to keep us afloat and cared for my siblings day-after-day, all while my mom and I battled cancer far from home. Every mile between us was another burden he carried alone, never allowing distance or exhaustion to weaken his resolve. While my mom stood at my bedside, my dad held the world together beyond it, bearing worry and fear without complaint. His strength was steady and unshakable, a foundation built on sacrifice and devotion.

Together, they formed a shield around me, absorbing the fear, the exhaustion, and the uncertainty so that I could focus on surviving. Their love did not cure me, but it carried me through every dark moment, every fragile hope, every step forward when giving up would have been easier. Even now, in their absence, I feel that love guiding me, reminding me that survival is rarely a solo act. It is built on the courage of those who stand beside us, fight for us, and believe in our lives even when the cost is great. This book is my way of remembering them, not only as parents, but as fierce warriors whose love made my survival possible.

I wrote this book for the doctors and nurses who fought for me in a time when medicine did not yet have all the answers. For the professionals who dared to hope alongside families, who tried new paths when old ones failed, who treated not just a disease, but a child. Their dedication reminds us that progress is built on courage, persistence, and belief in possibility.

I wrote this book for every survivor who has ever asked, "Why me?" For those who live with lasting effects, visible or invisible, and wonder what survival cost them. For those who feel guilty for being alive when others are not. For those who struggle to reconcile gratitude with grief. Survival is complicated. It is layered. It is not a finish line. It is a beginning that often comes with unanswered questions.

And I wrote this book for every family still in the fight. For those who feel exhausted, overwhelmed, and afraid. For those who need to hear, in the clearest possible way, "You are not alone." Even when it feels isolating. Even when the world moves on, you remain frozen in survival mode. Even when your strength feels gone. Someone else has stood where you stand now and lived to tell the story.

Most of all, I wrote this memoir to give meaning to the miracle I was given.

I lived for a reason. Not because I am special or stronger than others, but because survival itself carries purpose when we choose to seek it. That purpose does not have to be grand or public. It can be quiet. It can be found in compassion, in service, in listening, in simply being present for someone else's pain. Purpose is not about what we achieve. It is about what we do with what we've endured.

If you are reading this and carrying your own pain, whether from illness, loss, trauma, or heartbreak, I want you to know this: your suffering is not meaningless. It may not make sense yet. It may never fully make sense. But it does not disqualify you from hope. It does not erase your worth. And it does not mean your story ends here.

Tomorrow is still worth fighting for. Survival is not the end of the story. It is the invitation to write a new one. An invitation to decide how your pain will shape you, whether it will close your heart or open it wider. Whether it will silence you or give you a voice. Whether it will define you or deepen you.

This is my story, not just of surviving, but of choosing meaning.

And if it helps you take even one step toward finding purpose in your own pain, then the miracle continues. And that, perhaps, is the greatest survival of all.

# Epilogue

## The War on Childhood Cancer Continues
*from Tony and the Bell Asteri Foundation...*

In 1973, childhood cancer existed in a world that feels almost unrecognizable compared to today. In those days, hope was scarce, information was limited, and families faced unimaginable fear largely on their own. A diagnosis of childhood cancer then did not come with the vast resources, social workers assigned to guide parents, or networks of families who had walked the path before. There were no online forums, no Facebook groups, no late-night Google searches that could offer even a fragment of understanding. Parents received devastating news in sterile rooms and then were expected to somehow absorb it, process it, and move forward without a roadmap. For most childhood cancers, a diagnosis was less a fight and more a waiting period, because outcomes were so grim.

Survival rates were painfully low, treatments were experimental and brutal, and the emotional burden carried by families was often invisible and unsupported. There were no wish-granting organizations to give kids a joyful dream come true. No camps where young patients could feel normal, laugh freely, and meet others who understood without explanation. Siblings were largely forgotten casualties, expected to cope quietly while parents focused every ounce of energy on the child who was ill.

Parents missed work, drained savings, and made impossible choices without financial assistance, employer protections, or legislative safeguards. There was no federal framework recognizing childhood cancer as a distinct crisis worthy of focused funding and policy attention. Pain was endured privately, and grief was often borne in silence.

Progress since then has been extraordinary, but it is important to understand that progress is far more than better medicine. Yes, therapies have improved. Yes, survival rates for some cancers have risen dramatically. Acute lymphocytic leukemia, once almost universally fatal, now has a survival rate approaching 90%, a statistic that represents decades of research, clinical trials, courage, and sacrifice.

But survival statistics tell only part of the story. True progress means recognizing that childhood cancer affects entire families, not just individual patients. It means understanding that healing requires more than chemotherapy. It requires community, policy, compassion, and sustained investment.

Today, children with cancer are more likely to have access to multidisciplinary care teams that include social workers, child-life specialists, psychologists, and educators. Families are more likely to be connected with nonprofit organizations that provide financial aid, emotional support, and practical assistance. Camps exist where children with cancer and their siblings can experience joy without explanation, where scars and bald heads are normalized rather than questioned. Wish-granting programs offer moments of light in the darkest seasons, not because joy cures disease, but because it sustains the human spirit.

These advances matter deeply. They change how *families* survive, not just whether children do. And yet, despite all of this progress, the work is incomplete. Some legislation has begun to acknowledge childhood cancer through efforts such as the Childhood Cancer Data Initiative and select bills and policies that support federal research funding. These measures represent important steps forward, but they remain limited in scope and impact. Funding levels are still insufficient, many critical proposals fail to advance, and childhood cancer has yet to receive the sustained national attention and prioritization that the severity of the crisis demands.

While some childhood cancers now have hopeful outcomes, others remain devastatingly lethal. Pediatric brain cancers, in particular, continue to carry shockingly low survival rates, some nearly 100% fatal. For most of these diagnoses, treatment options have barely changed in decades. Children are still dying not because cures are impossible, but because research is underfunded, underprioritized, and undervalued. At the federal level, childhood cancer research receives only a small fraction of overall cancer funding, and that limited support must be stretched across all twelve major childhood cancer types and hundreds of subtypes. Despite this, cancer remains the leading cause of disease-related death among children. Rare pediatric cancers are especially overlooked, trapped in a system that prioritizes adult cancers with larger patient populations and more established advocacy infrastructures. This inequity is not accidental. It is structural.

Progress cannot be measured solely by what we have achieved. It must also be measured by what we have failed to do. Families today may have more support than they did in 1973, but too many still fall through the cracks. Financial toxicity remains a crushing burden. Parents still lose jobs, homes, and stability while trying to save their children. Mental health support is inconsistent and often inaccessible. Survivors face lifelong late effects with inadequate follow-up care and limited protections. And for families whose children do not survive, grief support remains uneven and insufficient.

We have come a long way from the isolating landscape of childhood cancer in 1973, but the distance traveled does not mean the destination has been reached. Better therapies save lives, but legislation sustains families. Research brings cures, but community restores dignity. Camps, scholarships, sibling programs, bereavement services, and advocacy efforts are not luxuries. They are essential components of a humane cancer care system. Childhood cancer is not just a medical crisis. It is a social one, a financial one, and a moral one.

The progress we celebrate today was made possible because people refused to accept the status quo of the past. The progress we still need will require that same refusal. Until every child, not just some, has a real chance at survival, until every family is supported before, during, and after diagnosis, until funding priorities reflect the urgency of young lives at stake, the work remains unfinished. Childhood cancer in 1973 taught us what happens when families are left alone. The future must prove that we learned from it.

*from Tony...*

Thank you for taking the time to read my story and to carry it with you. My hope does not end with these pages. I urge you to step forward and become a voice for the children and families who need one most. Childhood cancer demands more than sympathy. It requires action, advocacy, and collective resolve. In the pages that follow, you will find a list of organizations and institutions doing vital work within the childhood cancer community, along with meaningful ways you can stand beside them. You will also find practical, compassionate ways to support a family whose world has been shattered by a childhood cancer diagnosis. Even the smallest act can carry tremendous impact. Together, we can help ensure that no child and no family faces this fight alone.

Tony Garcia

# How You Can Help

$\mathcal{H}$elping children with cancer and their families requires far more than hope alone. It demands action. Consistent, compassionate, and practical action that recognizes both the medical reality of the disease and the emotional, financial, and logistical toll it takes on everyone in that child's life.

Childhood cancer does not affect only the child in treatment. It reshapes the daily life of parents, siblings, extended family, and caregivers. Truly helping means addressing the whole picture, from hospital rooms to living rooms, from policy decisions to dinner tables.

## ▶ Advocacy

One of the most powerful ways to help childhood cancer is through advocacy. Advocacy gives a voice to children who cannot speak for themselves and to families who are often too exhausted or overwhelmed to fight alone. Childhood cancer receives a disproportionately small share of research funding compared to adult cancers, despite being the leading cause of disease-related death in children.

Advocates help change this by raising awareness, educating lawmakers, supporting legislation for increased research funding, and pushing for safer, less toxic treatments. Advocacy can take many forms, including writing letters to representatives, participating in awareness walks, sharing survivor stories, or using social media to amplify the realities of childhood cancer. When people speak up collectively, awareness becomes action, and action becomes progress.

## ⟫ Fundraising

Raising funds is another essential pillar of support. Research saves lives, but research requires sustained financial investment. Fundraising efforts, whether large-scale charity events or small community-driven campaigns, help fund clinical trials, hospital programs, family support services, and survivor care. Fundraising also allows organizations to provide grants to families facing overwhelming expenses. Creative fundraisers, workplace donation drives, school events, benefit dinners, and online campaigns all contribute to a larger mission: giving children better chances and better futures.

Fundraising is not just about money. It is about engagement. It invites communities to participate, learn, and stand alongside families facing cancer.

## ⟫ Practical Help

Beyond advocacy and funding, practical help often makes the most immediate and meaningful difference in a family's daily life. Childhood cancer treatment is relentless. Parents juggle hospital stays, medications, appointments, and emotional care while trying to maintain some sense of normalcy.

Many families experience sudden financial strain due to lost income, travel costs, medical bills, and long hospital stays. Direct financial assistance, such as help with rent, utilities, gas cards, parking fees, or medical-related travel, can relieve an enormous burden. Even modest financial support can prevent families from having to choose between basic necessities and their child's care.

Support for siblings is another crucial and often overlooked need. Brothers and sisters of children with cancer frequently feel invisible as attention understandably centers on the child in treatment. Offering sibling childcare, covering costs for extracurricular activities, or arranging special outings helps siblings feel seen and valued. Providing tutoring or homework support during long hospital stays can also help siblings stay academically and emotionally grounded during a disruptive time.

Daily household tasks can quickly become overwhelming for families managing cancer. Offering home cleaning services or sending a maid removes a major stressor at a time when families are physically and emotionally drained. Clean homes contribute not only to comfort but also to health, especially for immunocompromised children. Similarly, lawn care or basic home maintenance can be invaluable, particularly for single-parent households or families spending most of their time at the hospital.

Acts of care that restore joy and dignity are just as important as meeting basic needs. Decorating a family's home for holidays, whether it's hanging lights, putting up a tree, or adding seasonal touches, can bring moments of celebration during an otherwise heavy season. These gestures remind families that joy is still possible, even in the midst of illness. They help preserve childhood experiences that cancer too often interrupts.

Food is another area where support has an immediate impact. Families frequently rely on hospital cafeterias or fast food during long treatment periods. Making meals, organizing meal trains, or purchasing gift cards for services like DoorDash gives families flexibility and nourishment without added effort. Gift cards allow parents to order food when schedules change unexpectedly, which is often the case during treatment.

Care packages thoughtfully assembled with comfort items, activities, snacks, or personal touches can brighten hospital stays and long days at home. For children, care packages may include toys, books, crafts, or games. For parents, they may include self-care items, coffee cards, journals, or warm blankets. Even small packages convey a powerful message: you are seen, and you are not alone.

Never underestimate the impact of writing cards, letters, or notes of encouragement. Words matter, especially during isolating hospital stays. A heartfelt card can offer hope on a difficult day or become something a child or parent holds onto long after treatment ends. Messages of encouragement, prayers, artwork from classmates, or notes from strangers all help families feel supported beyond their immediate circle.

Ultimately, helping overcome childhood cancer means showing up again and again in ways both large and small. It means advocating for systemic change while also folding laundry, mowing lawns, and sending meals. It means funding research for future cures while caring deeply for families navigating today's realities. Every act of support, whether public or private, contributes to a larger network of compassion that sustains families through one of the hardest journeys imaginable.

In summary...

When communities come together to advocate, fundraise, and offer practical help, they do more than ease burdens. They restore hope. And for children facing cancer and the families who love them, hope is not abstract. It is found in action, in kindness, and in the quiet assurance that they do not have to walk this path alone.

Tony Garcia

# From Hopelessness to Hope

*The Evolution of Childhood Cancer Treatment*

𝓘n the early twentieth century, a diagnosis of childhood cancer was almost universally fatal. For families in the 1940s, the word "leukemia" was not followed by treatment plans or survival statistics but by quiet preparation for loss. Doctors could offer comfort but little else. Children rarely lived more than weeks or months following a diagnosis. There were no proven therapies, no clinical trials as we know them today, and no expectation that science would soon change the outcome. Yet within that bleak reality, the seeds of transformation were being planted.

The 1940s marked the dawn of chemotherapy and the first glimmer of hope in childhood cancer treatment. In 1947, Dr. Sidney Farber, often called the "father of modern chemotherapy," reported something previously unimaginable: temporary remission in children with leukemia. Using aminopterin, a folic acid antagonist, Farber was able to slow the uncontrolled growth of leukemia cells. The remissions were partial and brief. Most children relapsed, but the significance was profound. For the first time, cancer had responded to a drug. Leukemia was no longer entirely untouchable. It was a small crack in what had always been an unbreakable wall.

During these early years, researchers also began to distinguish between different types of leukemia. Acute lymphoblastic leukemia (ALL) emerged as a disease that, while still deadly, showed more responsiveness to early chemotherapy than other forms. This differentiation was crucial. It allowed scientists to ask more precise questions and design more targeted experiments, laying the groundwork for future progress.

In the early 1950s, most children with leukemia were not dying from cancer progression alone. They were bleeding to death. Leukemia destroys the body's ability to produce healthy platelets, the blood components responsible for clotting. Without platelets, children developed uncontrollable internal bleeding and hemorrhages from even minor injuries. At that time, there was no effective way to replace platelets. As a result, many children died within days or weeks of diagnosis, often before doctors could even attempt chemotherapy. The disease progressed faster than medicine could respond, and treatment itself was frequently impossible because patients could not survive long enough to receive it.

Dr. Emil Freireich transformed this grim reality. Working at the National Cancer Institute, Freireich recognized that stopping bleeding was not a secondary concern, but it was essential to survival. He pioneered the use of platelet transfusions from fresh blood, demonstrating that restoring platelets could control hemorrhaging and stabilize children long enough to undergo treatment. This insight fundamentally changed leukemia care. For the first time, doctors could keep patients alive while chemotherapy did its work.

To make platelet transfusion feasible on a larger scale, Freireich partnered with engineer George Judson to develop the first continuous-flow blood cell separator. This groundbreaking machine allowed platelets to be efficiently collected from donors while returning the remaining blood components to the donor, making repeated and reliable platelet transfusions possible. The technology became a cornerstone of modern blood banking and cancer care and remains essential to this day.

By addressing the immediate, life-threatening problem of bleeding, Freireich made chemotherapy viable for children with leukemia. His work did not stop there. He was also a key architect of combination chemotherapy, advancing the idea that multiple drugs used together could overcome cancer's resistance mechanisms. This dual breakthrough, including supportive care that kept children alive and combination therapy that targeted leukemia aggressively, helped convert what had been a certain death sentence into a disease that could be treated and, increasingly, cured.

Dr. Freireich's contributions reshaped pediatric oncology at its foundation. He proved that curing cancer required more than powerful drugs. It required supporting the body through the fight. By stopping children from bleeding to death and enabling sustained treatment, he changed not only survival rates but the very possibility of a cure.

Through the 1960s, researchers learned even more about how ineffective a single drug would be. Cancer adapted quickly, and remissions achieved with one agent were often short-lived. Researchers began experimenting more and more with combination chemotherapy, using multiple drugs with different mechanisms of action to attack cancer cells on several fronts at once. Drugs such as vincristine, prednisone, and mercaptopurine became cornerstones of treatment. This approach dramatically improved outcomes for children with ALL, extending survival and, for some, achieving long-term remission.

At the same time, doctors recognized that saving children from cancer required more than killing cancer cells. The toxicity of chemotherapy was severe, and many children died not from cancer itself but from infections or organ failure caused by treatment. This reality led to major advances in supportive care. The development of antibiotics, improved nutritional support, and safer hospital environments allowed children to survive the rigors of aggressive treatment. Supportive care quietly became as essential as chemotherapy itself, transforming once-lethal side effects into manageable risks.

The 1970s ushered in an era of rapid progress and intensified treatment. Armed with growing confidence and better supportive care, researchers adopted a more aggressive philosophy. Multi-drug regimens became standard, and treatment protocols grew longer and more complex. This decade saw sharp declines in childhood cancer mortality, not only for leukemia but also for lymphomas and certain bone cancers. The prevailing belief was that more intensive therapy would produce better outcomes and, in many cases, it did.

Just as important was a shift in thinking. Cancer was increasingly understood as a systemic disease, even when it appeared localized. This insight justified prolonged and comprehensive treatment approaches, ensuring that microscopic disease was eradicated. What had once been considered experimental was becoming standardized, and childhood cancer care began to take shape as a coordinated, research-driven discipline.

By the 1980s and 1990s, the focus shifted from simply increasing intensity to refining protocols. Large cooperative groups conducted serial clinical trials designed to answer specific questions. Which drugs were essential? When should they be given? How much treatment was enough, and how much was too much? Studies such as CCG 1922 introduced concepts like delayed intensification and demonstrated that early response to therapy, particularly bone marrow response in ALL, could predict outcomes.

This era also introduced risk stratification, a transformative concept in pediatric oncology. Children were grouped into risk categories based on factors such as age, white blood cell count, genetics, and treatment response. Therapy could then be tailored accordingly, reducing toxicity for those likely to do well, while intensifying treatment for those at higher risk of relapse. This personalized approach improved survival while beginning to address the growing concern about treatment-related harm.

By the 2000s, the impact of decades of research was unmistakable. Five-year survival rates for childhood ALL exceeded 85%, a staggering contrast to the zero survival rate of the 1940s. Overall survival for childhood cancers rose dramatically, though disparities remained. Certain cancers, including some central nervous system tumors and high-risk solid tumors, continued to present major challenges.

As survival improved, a new reality emerged. Childhood cancer was no longer only about saving lives, but it was also about protecting futures. The growing population of survivors revealed the long-term consequences of treatment, including heart disease, secondary cancers, endocrine disorders, cognitive challenges, and chronic health conditions. These late effects became a central concern, shifting research priorities toward treatments that cure without causing lifelong harm.

Today's research is guided by molecular insights and precision medicine. Scientists now study minimal residual disease (MRD) to detect tiny amounts of cancer cells invisible under a microscope, allowing therapy to be adjusted with remarkable accuracy. Genetic and molecular profiling is helping identify targeted therapies designed to be more effective and less toxic than traditional chemotherapy.

The overarching story of childhood cancer treatment is one of extraordinary progress born from collaboration, persistence, and courage. What was once a uniformly fatal diagnosis has become, for many children, a survivable and even curable disease. This transformation did not happen overnight, nor did it come without cost. It was achieved through decades of clinical trials, brave patients and families, relentless researchers, and a comprehensive care model that treats not just the disease, but the child as a whole.

Yet the story is far from finished. Survival alone is no longer enough. We must focus on ensuring that children who survive cancer can live full, healthy lives long after treatment ends. The journey from hopelessness to hope has changed the landscape of pediatric medicine, and it continues, driven by the belief that every child deserves not just to survive, but to thrive.

In the United States, approximately 1,800 children die of cancer every year. Globally, more than 100,000 children die of cancer every year. Although childhood cancer is considered "rare," it does not seem so rare when you look at the actual numbers. In 2026, it is expected that more than 400,000 kids will be diagnosed with cancer around the world. And although much progress has been made for certain cancers, we are failing miserably for many others. It is long past time to do something.

Cancer has waged war on our children.

**We stand ready to fight!**

# Main Childhood Cancer Types

- Leukemia: Most common, affecting white blood cells (e.g., ALL, AML).

- Brain & CNS Tumors: Cancers in the brain and spinal cord (e.g., Astrocytoma, DIPG).

- Lymphoma: Cancers of the lymphatic system (Hodgkin & Non-Hodgkin).

- Neuroblastoma: Nerve tissue cancer, common in infants.

- Wilms Tumor: Kidney cancer in young children.

- Bone Cancer: Tumors in bone (e.g., Osteosarcoma, Ewing sarcoma).

- Soft Tissue Sarcomas: Cancers in muscle, fat, or other tissues (e.g., Rhabdomyosarcoma).

- Retinoblastoma: Eye cancer.

- Liver Tumors: Cancers of the liver (e.g., Hepatoblastoma).

- Germ Cell Tumors: Develop from reproductive cells (e.g., in gonads, brain).

- Kidney Tumors: Beyond Wilms, other kidney cancers.

- Other Carcinomas & Melanomas: Rare in children, but include skin cancers and other epithelial tumors.

# Childhood Cancer Legislation & Policy

*The following are examples of legislation and policies that have helped to advance childhood cancer outcomes. The childhood cancer community needs more allies. We urge you to get involved in advocacy.*

**Childhood Cancer Data Initiative (CCDI)**

A federal data-sharing initiative to improve pediatric cancer research by collecting and integrating clinical and research data nationwide.

Purpose & goals:

- Better understanding of pediatric cancer biology, treatment, survivorship, and prevention.
- Enable researchers and clinicians to access shared data to accelerate discoveries.
- Promote standardized data collection across institutions.

The CCDI is funded and ongoing through authorization and appropriations (e.g., included in appropriations tied to STAR Act funding).

Why it matters:

By consolidating data, CCDI aims to help researchers identify new treatment targets and improve outcomes for children and AYAs (adolescents and young adults) with cancer.

## Gabriella Miller Kids First Research Act & Kids First Research Act 2.0 (GMKF)

Named after Gabriella Miller, a young childhood cancer advocate who died from a rare brain tumor, this law redirects funds (originally set aside for political party conventions) into pediatric research.

Original Act (2014)

- Established a 10-year pediatric research initiative administered through NIH's Common Fund.
- Authorized about $126 million over the decade for pediatric research, especially focusing on genetics and disease mechanisms.

Kids First Research Act 2.0

- Reauthorizes the Kids First program (through FY2028).
- Strengthens coordination of pediatric research at NIH and improves reporting requirements to Congress.
- Became Public Law in Jan 2025.

Program outcomes:

- Supports the Kids First Data Resource Center, which aggregates whole-genome sequencing and clinical data to understand childhood cancers and congenital anomalies.

Why it matters:

This legislation creates a major genetic and clinical data platform used by researchers worldwide, boosting discoveries about pediatric cancers.

**STAR Act** (Survivorship, Treatment, Access, and Research Act)

A comprehensive pediatric cancer law signed in 2018 and reauthorized in 2023.

<u>Core components</u>:

- Strengthens pediatric cancer research funding and programs.
- Expands and improves childhood cancer surveillance via enhanced cancer registry capabilities.
- Promotes research on long-term effects of childhood cancer treatment.
- Supports initiatives addressing quality of life for survivors.

<u>Reauthorization</u>:

- In January 2023, Congress reauthorized the STAR Act, continuing its programs through FY2028.

<u>Why it matters</u>:

STAR is considered the most comprehensive federal childhood cancer law, addressing research, treatment, and survivor support.

**Research to Accelerate Cures and Equity (RACE) for Children Act**

A law passed in 2017 as part of the FDA Reauthorization Act and fully implemented in 2020. It amends the Pediatric Research Equity Act (PREA).

<u>Purpose</u>:

Ensure that new cancer drugs developed for adults with targets relevant to pediatric cancers are studied in children.

<u>Under RACE</u>:

- FDA can require pediatric studies for drugs with molecular targets relevant to childhood cancers.

- Eliminates exemptions that previously allowed sponsors to avoid pediatric evaluation of cancer drugs.

Impact:

- Significantly increases the number of oncology drugs subject to pediatric study requirements.
- Encourages earlier pediatric evaluation and potential labeling of cancer therapies for children.

Why it matters:

Before RACE, many targeted therapies were developed for adults with little or no pediatric data. This act helps close that gap.

## Pediatric Research Equity Act (PREA)

A 2007 FDA law that allows FDA to require pediatric studies of drugs when appropriate. It was later amended by RACE (above) to strengthen pediatric oncology requirements.

Core points:

- Requires pediatric assessments for new drugs unless a waiver or deferral is granted.
- Works with the Best Pharmaceuticals for Children Act (BPCA), which offers incentives for voluntary pediatric studies.

Relation to RACE:

RACE amended PREA to eliminate the "orphan drug" exemption and make pediatric cancer drug studies more likely.

**Mikaela Naylon Give Kids a Chance Act**

Legislative efforts focused on incentivizing pediatric drug development and expanding access to therapies.

- Creating Hope Act (2011): Established the Priority Review Voucher (PRV) program for companies developing treatments for rare pediatric diseases.
- Give Kids a Chance Act: Combines the original Give Kids a Chance and Creating Hope Reauthorization, expanding PRV use and authorizing pediatric combination therapy studies.

Why it matters:

PRVs and similar incentives help overcome weak market incentives for pediatric drug development, stimulating research for rare childhood conditions.

**Congressional Childhood Cancer Caucus**

The Congressional Childhood Cancer Caucus was founded in 2009 by Representative Michael McCaul (TX-10) and Representative Chris Van Hollen to aid members of Congress in working together to address pediatric cancer. They raise awareness, advocate in support of measures to prevent the pain, suffering, and long-term effects of childhood cancers, and work toward the goal of eliminating cancer as a threat to all children. Visit the website to learn more, and we urge you to get involved in advocacy:

childhoodcancer-mccaul.house.gov

# Organizations & Resources

- **Blood Cancer United** (Formerly, the Leukemia & Lymphoma Society): bloodcancerunited.org

- **MD Anderson Cancer Center**: mdanderson.org

- **Gold Together for Childhood Cancer, American Cancer Society**: acsresources.org/property/goldtogether

- **CureFest for Childhood Cancer**: curefest.com

- **Rally Foundation for Childhood Cancer Research**: rallyfoundation.org

- **Coalition Against Childhood Cancer**: cac2.org

- **Congressional Childhood Cancer Caucus**: childhoodcancer-mccaul.house.gov

- **Alliance for Childhood Cancer** : allianceforchildhoodcancer.org

- **American Cancer Society Cancer Action Network** (ACS CAN): fightcancer.org

- **Children's Cancer Cause**: childrenscancercause.org

- **Children's Oncology Group**: childrensoncologygroup.org

- **National Institutes of Health**: nih.gov

- **National Cancer Institute**: cancer.gov

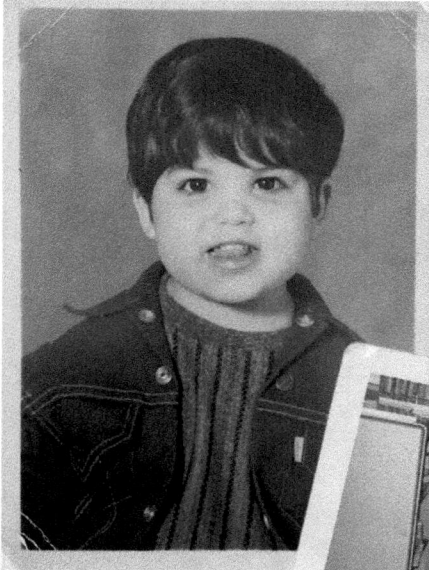

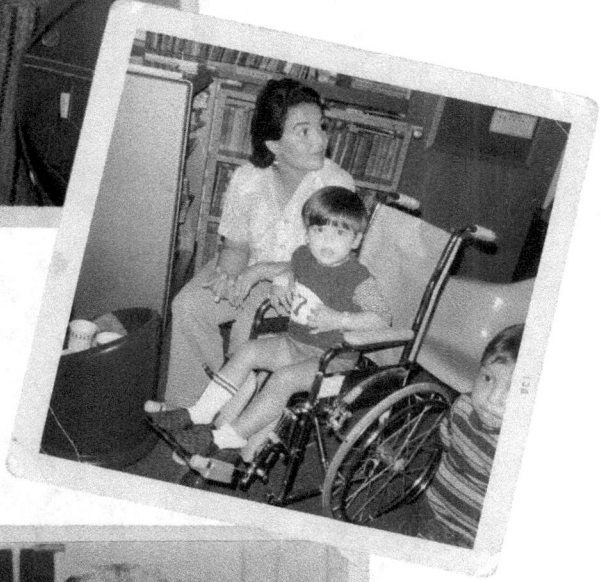

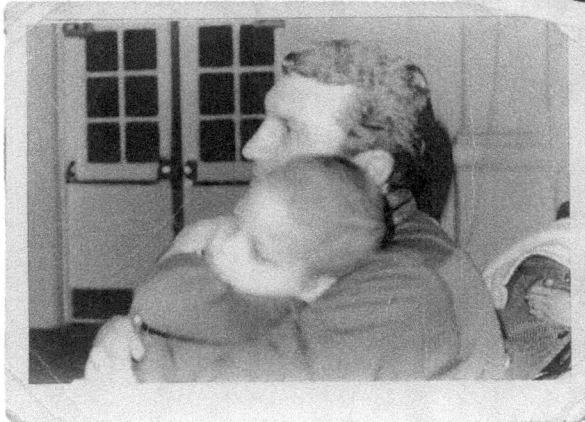

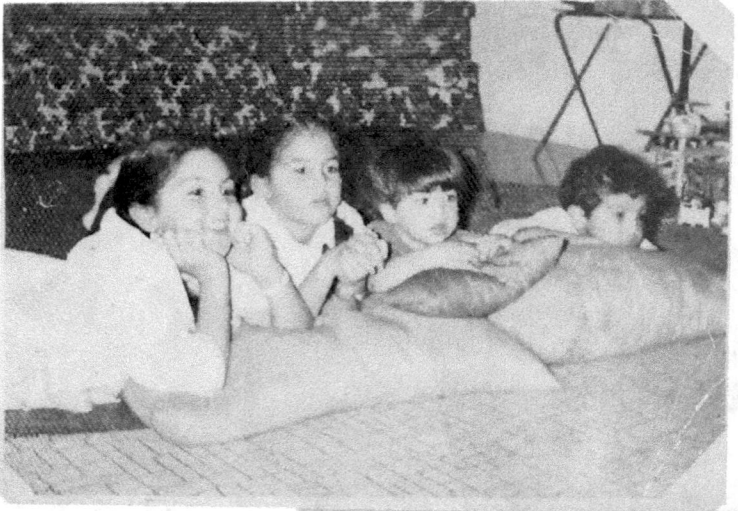

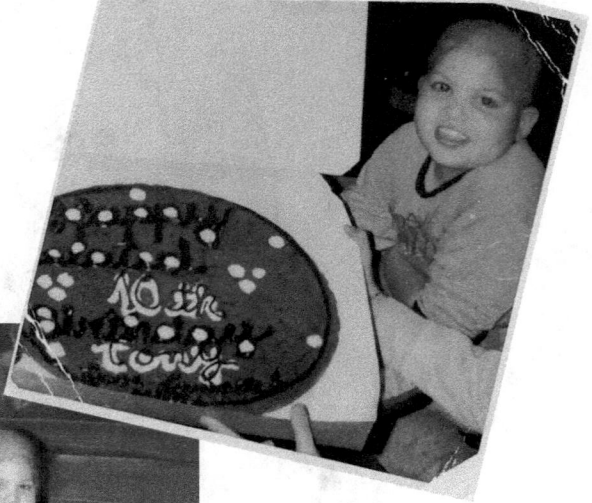

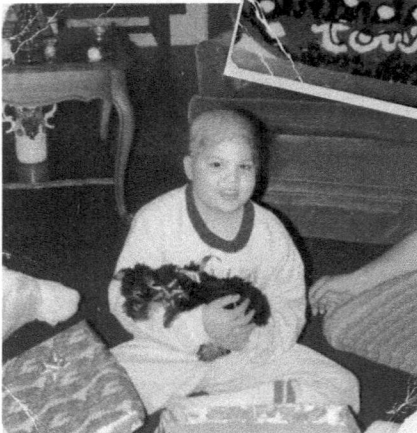

Find more resources at
www.bellasteri.com

www.ingramcontent.com/pod-product-compliance
Lightning Source LLC
Chambersburg PA
CBHW070813280326
41934CB00012B/3184